THE LITTLE BOOK OF
CHAKRAS

THE LITTLE BOOK OF CHAKRAS

An Hachette UK Company
www.hachette.co.uk

Summersdale Publishers Ltd
Part of Octopus Publishing Group Limited
Carmelite House
50 Victoria Embankment
LONDON
EC4Y 0DZ
UK

www.summersdale.com

Printed and bound in Poland

ISBN: 978-1-78783-685-3

DISCLAIMER
The author and the publisher cannot accept responsibility for any misuse or misunderstanding of any information contained herein, or any loss, damage or injury, be it health, financial or otherwise, suffered by any individual or group acting upon or relying on information contained herein. None of the views or suggestions in this book is intended to replace medical opinion from a doctor who is familiar with your particular circumstances. If you have concerns about your health, please seek professional advice.

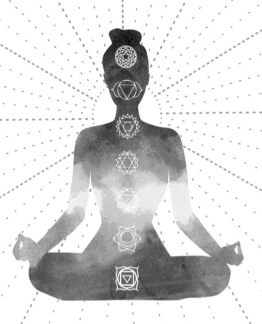

THE LITTLE BOOK OF
CHAKRAS

ELSIE WILD

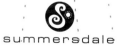

summersdale

CONTENTS

INTRODUCTION

Chakras have always existed but have become increasingly popular in recent years with the rise of New Age wellness retreats. You've probably heard chakras mentioned in passing, maybe at your yoga class, or on social media. You may have seen the word on jewellery or bottles of essential oils along with the phrase "this is great for your chakras", but what does that really mean? What are chakras? And why should you care about them?

If you've ever been just a little bit curious about chakras but have no idea where to begin, you've come to the right place. This book will be your basic guide to the seven main chakras in the system, from the root to the crown. Inside these pages you will learn which crystals, essential oils, yoga poses, mantras and affirmations work best to open and balance specific chakras.

While the chakra system originated from sacred Hindu texts, people from all backgrounds and religions have embraced the benefits of chakra healing and have experienced improved overall health and well-being. You don't have to be religious to practise anything in this book – just remember to always be mindful and

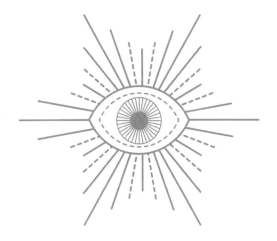

respectful when practising anything from a culture that isn't your own.

It's important to remember that this is just an introduction to the subject; you can discover the essentials in these pages and delve deeper into the world of chakras through further reading, if you wish – it's your own personal journey, whatever that may look like for you.

Let's get started!

WHAT ARE CHAKRAS?

The word *chakra* comes from the Sanskrit word, *cakra*, which translates to "wheel" or "disc". Essentially, chakras are spinning wheels of *prana*, Sanskrit for life-force, which circulate energy to certain parts of our bodies. When all of our chakras are open and aligned, prana can move freely, and the mind, body and spirit are in perfect harmony.

There are seven chakras that run from the base of the spine to the top of the head. Each has its own physical function and emotional and spiritual aspects. If something feels off, like you have an ache or a pain, it could be that one of your chakras is blocked and therefore out of balance, or alignment, with the rest of the body. Unblocking and rebalancing your chakra can help you to feel well again. However, too much energy flowing into one chakra can make it overactive, which can cause burnout, hyperactivity, or stress. To be balanced, energy must flow through the chakras equally.

A BRIEF HISTORY OF CHAKRAS

The chakra network derived from a complex and ancient belief system that has existed for thousands of years, originating in Ancient India. They were first mentioned in the Vedas – the sacred scriptures of Hinduism – dating from the period 1500 to 100 BCE. However, the chakra system may have existed for much longer than this, given that most spiritual teachings were passed down orally from teacher to student before being recorded in writing.

Chakras were mentioned in the later Vedic Sanskrit text called the Upanishads, which roughly translates to "at the foot of the teacher". Along with chakras, the Upanishads discuss meditation, philosophy and spiritual knowledge.

In early Sanskrit texts, chakras were viewed as "meditative visualizations" that combined flowers and mantras. In later writings, chakras were considered points of prana that connected the physical and spiritual energy channels.

Kundalini yoga, a physical and spiritual practice from the Upanishads, also had a hand in the development of the chakra knowledge system. Kundalini is a form of primal energy that is coiled at the base of the spine, like a snake. It typically lies dormant unless awoken by physical activity, such as yoga, breathing exercises, visualizations, mantras and mudras (symbolic hand gestures used in yoga or meditation). When awake, the kundalini can "turn on" all your chakras at the same time, though it may take years and lots of practice to wake up the kundalini. Kundalini yoga teaches us that true enlightenment comes from within. Once the chakras wake up, they have a positive effect on the body and spirit, including improved health, vitality, and mental clarity, among other benefits.

While the chakra system originated from ancient Hindu texts, the idea of energy centres has existed throughout history in many cultures, including the Egyptians, Chinese, Sufis, Greeks, Incas, Mayans, and the indigenous tribes of North America.

THE CHAKRA SYSTEM

It has been said that there are as many as 114 chakras in the body, but we'll be going over the seven main chakras in the chakra system, and a few others at the end of this book.

The number of chakras in the system differs depending on the belief system you follow. Buddhist texts mention five chakras, while Hindu texts mention seven. We'll be discussing seven chakras, as it is the most commonly agreed-upon system.

The major chakras are located along the spine, starting from the base and rising to the top of the head. Each one represents a different area in your life and has specific requirements that must be fulfilled to be balanced. Think of the chakras as a type of spiritual nervous system that keeps your prana moving steadily throughout the body.

The lower chakras – the root chakra, the sacral chakra and the solar plexus chakra – represent the physical and emotional needs that keep us grounded to the earth and the physical realm. The upper chakras – the throat chakra, the third eye chakra and the crown chakra – are regarded as the spiritual centres; these act as access points to our highest streams of consciousness. The heart chakra rests in the middle, connecting the physical realm with the spiritual realm.

Every living thing has a chakra system, from your precious pet to the tree in your garden, because everything in life is made out of energy. To be healthy, we must keep our chakras healthy and balanced at all times.

WORKING WITH YOUR CHAKRAS

There are many ways to harness the power of your chakras and keep them balanced, open and unblocked. These include classic methods like meditation, yoga, visualizations, mantras, mudras and feeding your chakras. We will also be discussing popular methods of crystal healing and essential oils. It may be that only some of these approaches work for you, or that some work for one chakra but not for another. You can also receive outside help with your chakras by going to a reiki session, doing acupuncture, attending yoga classes, or seeing a dietician.

It's important to remember as you go through this book that you won't be able to open your chakras in just one day; it takes time, practice and focus to see results. Don't be discouraged if you don't feel a difference right away.

ROOT CHAKRA

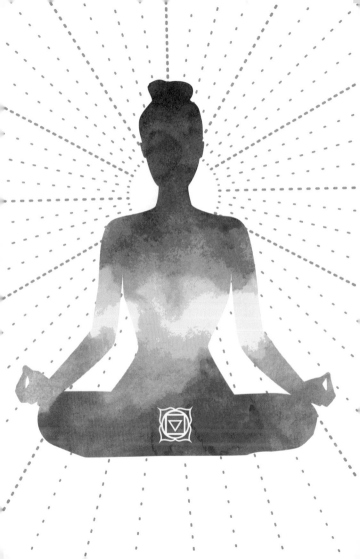

OVERVIEW

The root chakra, also known as muladhara, is the foundation on which our souls and spiritual energies are built. Located at the base of the spine, near the tailbone, the root chakra centres on our survival instinct and need for security. It is also associated with our personal strengths, willpower, self-esteem and passions. When it's balanced, we are grounded, energetic and independent. When unbalanced, we become fearful, unstable and insecure. Do not take the root chakra for granted as it is the base of our mental and physical health and well-being, helping us to keep our feet firmly on the ground.

KEY FACTS

Sanskrit: Muladhara – *mula* means "root" and *adhara* means "base"
Colour: Red
Element: Earth
Planet: Saturn
Zodiac sign: Capricorn & Aquarius
Motto: "I am"

MENTAL AND PHYSICAL ASPECTS

As the first chakra, muladhara is the centre of our physical and mental health. If we have an issue in our lives, be it medical, mental or spiritual, it's worth checking this chakra first to get to the "root" of the problem.

The root chakra rules the legs, feet and bones, but also deals with our sense of smell. When the root chakra is unbalanced, it can manifest itself physically in lower-back and foot pain, sciatica, constipation, varicose veins, haemorrhoids, osteoarthritis and immune-related disorders.

If the root chakra is unbalanced, you may unconsciously clench your muscles, like you are bracing for impact. This is because the root chakra deals with our "fight-or-flight" response. When our root chakra is balanced, we feel energetic, well rested and graceful on our feet. Our bones are strong, and we are at ease in our bodies and with the world.

The root chakra is in tune with our core needs for survival (food, water, shelter and security), which is why it is at the centre of our mental and emotional health. When these needs are met, we feel confident, powerful, strong, independent and brave.

If our root chakra is unbalanced, it is likely that our basic needs are not being met. Our survival instincts are in overdrive and we cannot focus on much else. This lack of stability creates fear, insecurity, low self-esteem and co-dependency. People can also start to suffer from anxiety, depression and panic attacks.

The root chakra may be the most important chakra – if we're without a stable foundation it's difficult to do anything else.

THE ACHE FOR
HOME LIVES
IN ALL OF US,
THE SAFE PLACE
WHERE WE CAN
GO AS WE ARE
AND NOT BE
QUESTIONED.

MAYA ANGELOU

FOOD AND DIET

What we feed our bodies is what we feed our chakras, so if we want to keep a particular chakra healthy and clean, we need to give it the right foods. To nourish your root chakra, it's good to give it root vegetables, and not just because of the shared name. Root vegetables absorb high amounts of vitamins and nutrients. Some great choices are sweet potatoes, carrots, turnips, garlic, parsnips, onions, swede, ginger and turmeric.

Protein-rich foods are great for the root chakra to build strong muscles and bones. Choices like eggs, beans, peanut butter, nuts and lean meat can really satisfy muladhara.

Lastly, because the first chakra is red, it's good to feed it red foods like apples, beets, tomatoes, pomegranates, strawberries and raspberries to match the colour and energy.

CRYSTALS

Crystals that are associated with the root chakra, and help heal, clean and stimulate it, include:

Haematite: grounding, manifestation and focus.
Jasper: grounding, cleansing and calm.
Jet: support, protection and harmony.
Obsidian: self-reflection, growth and protection.
Onyx: protection, calm and release.
Ruby: passion, protection and prosperity.
Smoky Quartz: healing, grounding and letting go.
Tiger's Eye: good fortune, prosperity and inspiration.
Tourmaline: cleansing, grounding and protection.

Use these crystals during meditation as you try to open your root chakra. You can also keep a crystal in your pocket throughout the day to feel the effects more frequently, or when you need a little boost of self-confidence.

ESSENTIAL OILS

Essential oils are a great tool because they have so many different uses. You can use them during chakra work – while meditating or practising yoga, for example – to help open and balance muladhara. They can also be utilized while relaxing, or when you want to feel grounded. Here are a few oils associated with the root chakra:

Cedar: balance, steadiness, protection and purity.
Clove: love, money, protection and drive.
Ginger: abundance, liberation and success.
Patchouli: connection, stimulation and money.
Rosemary: healing, protection and uplifted spirit.
Sandalwood: healing, protection and peace.
Vetiver: calming, grounding and protection.

WHEN THE ROOTS ARE DEEP, THERE IS NO REASON TO FEAR THE WIND.

AFRICAN PROVERB

YOGA POSES

One of the best ways to open and realign your chakras is by doing yoga. Yoga balances the body – physically, mentally and spiritually. When we do yoga, we become more connected with the body and our chakras. For muladhara, it's important to focus on yoga poses that move your spine and legs, helping you become grounded. Here are a few poses to try out:

Warrior I (Virabhadrasana I): A popular pose that's perfect for beginners, this is a standing yoga pose that helps improve balance and stability, while encouraging bodily awareness. This pose strengthens the legs, feet, core and back.

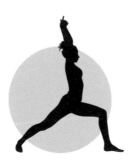

Tree Pose (Vrikshasana): A staple in many yoga routines, this is a balancing pose that strengthens the legs and feet to help you feel steady and grounded. It also straightens the spine to boost self-esteem.

Triangle Pose (Trikonasana): This is a standing yoga pose that helps tone and strengthen the legs and inner thighs while increasing stability and decreasing stress. It also relieves lower-back pain. If you need to feel empowered, give this pose a try.

Eagle Pose (Garudasana): The eagle pose is a standing position that will improve your balance over time. This pose will help you strengthen your calves, ankles, thighs and core. It will improve your concentration and can also relieve back pain and sciatica.

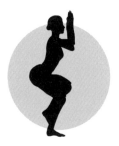

Exercise Tip

Do yoga, or any physical activity, outside if you can. The root chakra is associated with the earth and rules the feet, so if you walk or do yoga barefoot, you'll feel more connected with the earth and with your root chakra.

MEDITATION AND AFFIRMATIONS

When it comes to healing your chakras, meditation can create a safe space to find calm and get grounded. If you feel like your root chakra is blocked, try this simple meditation:

 Step One: Find a quiet spot, preferably outdoors. Stand up straight with your feet apart and knees slightly bent, placing your weight evenly on the soles of your bare feet.

 Step Two: Close your eyes and take a few deep, slow breaths.

 Step Three: In your mind, picture a red glow at the base of your spine. Visualize that glow slowly expanding, making the area warm and relaxed.

 Step Four: Place your hands out in front of you with the palms up, and have your thumbs touch your ring fingers to form circles. This is the Prithivi Mudra, associated with centring the spirit. Slowly start chanting the *lam* mantra (pronounced "lahm").

 Step Five: When you're ready, open your eyes and rest for a moment before continuing with the rest of your day.

Words are powerful. They can shape our mindset and comfort us in times of crisis. Affirmations can be particularly effective at giving us emotional support and confidence. When dealing with the root chakra, we need to remind ourselves that we are safe and strong. Below is a list of affirmations to help unblock the root chakra and restore balance. Repeat these in your head, like a mantra, as you meditate, or during times of fear and uncertainty. You can also write them down to keep on hand when you need encouragement.

- "I am grounded and present in my life."
- "My needs will be met."
- "I recognize the love that surrounds me in all of its forms."
- "I feel deeply rooted."
- "I feel safe and secure."
- "I trust myself."
- "I'm standing up for my values."

Feel free to create your own affirmations – just remember to focus on stability, confidence, courage and security when composing them.

SACRAL
CHAKRA

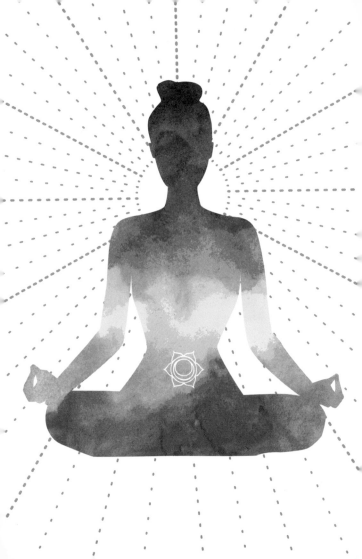

OVERVIEW

Once our root chakra is open and our basic needs are met, the fun can really start. We're now in the perfect position to explore the wonders and magic of life. Located just below the navel, the sacral chakra, or svadisthana, rules over sexuality, creativity, connection and physical activity. It allows us to experience the world through our senses and emotions, making them that much more intense and pleasurable. When this chakra is balanced, we can enjoy all the pleasures life has to offer. We vibrate with joy and can connect to others with authentic, healthy emotions. When unbalanced, we become guilt-ridden, creatively blocked and unable to express our emotions and desires.

KEY FACTS

Sanskrit: Svadisthana – "where you are being established"
Colour: Orange
Element: Water
Planet: Jupiter
Zodiac sign: Sagittarius & Pisces
Motto: "I feel"

MENTAL AND PHYSICAL ASPECTS

Svadisthana is located in the lower abdomen and represents our reproductive organs, as well as the kidneys, bladder, pelvis and spleen. It keeps things flowing regularly, which makes sense, given that it is ruled by water.

The sacral chakra is very active, which in turn makes us want to run, jump and generally get physical. For this chakra to stay healthy, it needs to stay hydrated as we are constantly doing activities that cause us to lose liquids, such as sweating and urinating.

When this chakra is balanced, we are always on the go, our sexual appetite is healthy and everything is moving in harmony. When the sacral chakra is unbalanced, we may see it physically in sexual dysfunction, chronic lower-back pain, arthritis, hip issues, and bladder problems. If svadisthana is blocked, it could mean that our needs are not being met – for example, not getting enough liquids or enough sex.

The sacral chakra is our pleasure centre – not just because it rules over reproductive organs, but because it's where we experience everything that makes life worthwhile: connecting with others, expressing ourselves creatively, feeling joy, eating good food and feeling good in our bodies. In the root chakra, we were trying to survive; in the sacral chakra, we are trying to live.

This chakra feels emotions instantly and intensely. When balanced, we can express our emotions in healthy ways. When unbalanced we ignore those feelings or express them in unhealthy ways, be it obsession, mood swings, or through controlling, clingy or unemotional behaviour. We need to be able to have healthy outlets through which to express our feelings in order to be happy. When we don't have an outlet, we can become creatively blocked, depressed, or stagnant emotionally.

In order to keep svadisthana balanced and open, make sure your emotional needs are being met: hang out with friends, be comfortable in your sexuality and express yourself creatively.

LET'S NOT FORGET
THAT THE LITTLE
EMOTIONS ARE
THE GREAT
CAPTAINS OF
OUR LIVES
AND WE OBEY
THEM WITHOUT
REALIZING IT.

VINCENT VAN GOGH

FOOD AND DIET

With the constant energy that svadisthana keeps exerting, it's essential to keep this chakra nourished. Most importantly, the sacral chakra should be hydrated at all times. Svadisthana is associated with water and rules over the kidneys and the bladder, so it's vital to maintain a steady intake of water. Coconut water, herbal teas, and good old H_2O are excellent choices along with various types of melon for their high water content. Try to avoid caffeine as it can overstimulate this chakra, and it's already energetic enough.

Foods rich in omega-3, like salmon, trout, flax, almond, walnut, pumpkin and sesame seeds, are all great options as they reduce inflammation. Foods like pomegranate and strawberries are also great to stimulate sex drive.

Lastly, you can't go wrong with eating orange foods like mangoes, oranges, carrots, sweet potatoes, honey, orange peppers, peaches and apricots.

CRYSTALS

Crystals that are associated with the sacral chakra, and help heal, clean and stimulate it, include:

Amber: concentration, purification and health.
Calcite: energy, wisdom and bravery.
Carnelian: motivation, endurance and courage.
Citrine: joy, creativity and abundance.
Fire Agate: protection, awareness and drive.
Lemon Quartz: structure, focus and communication.
Moonstone: stability, spirituality and sensuality.
Sunstone: healing, happiness and warmth.
Tiger's Eye: good fortune, prosperity and inspiration.

Use these crystals to open your sacral chakra during meditation, or wear these crystals in a pocket close to your abdomen to bring it closer to svadisthana. Perhaps take a healing bath with them to boost feelings of confidence, especially right before a big event.

ESSENTIAL OILS

Here are a few essential oils that help open the sacral chakra and promote feelings of self-acceptance and pleasure:

Bergamot: balance, joy, strength, understanding and success.

Cardamom: clarity, courage, enthusiasm, wisdom and love.

Geranium: balance, tranquility, health, protection and self-assurance.

Grapefruit: confidence, intelligence, creativity, mental clarity and emotional openness.

Neroli: calmness, happiness, peace, money and gentleness.

Orange: creativity, cheer, positivity, luck and divination.

Ylang-Ylang: self-confidence, understanding, enthusiasm, uplifting energies and a spiritual awakening.

Tip: Place a few drops of diluted essential oil on your lower back to open and stimulate the chakra. Or use massage oil with the scents mentioned above to get the full effect.

OFTEN THE HANDS
WILL SOLVE A
MYSTERY THAT
THE INTELLECT
HAS STRUGGLED
WITH IN VAIN.

CARL JUNG

YOGA POSES

For the sacral chakra, it's important to focus on strengthening your core muscles and to keep your body moving to simulate the flow of creativity. While you can boost your sacral chakra with your own yoga moves, here are a few poses to try out:

Seated Forward Bend (Paschimottanasana): A basic stretch for the lower back and hamstrings. This pose stretches the spine and shoulders while also stimulating the liver and kidneys, as well as calming both body and mind. This serves as a great warm-up and can be calming at the end of your routine.

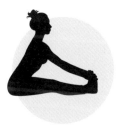

Garland Pose (Mālāsana):
A beginner level squat that
strengthens the lower body while
opening the hips, ankles, groin
and the Achilles. This pose
improves balance, digestion,
memory and concentration,
while also helping with
sex drive.

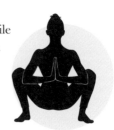

Bridge Pose (Setu Bandha Sarvangasana):
A backbend pose that opens the hips and pelvic
area while stimulating and opening the sacral
chakra. This pose helps strengthen the hamstrings,
quadriceps and hips. It also helps with stress, mild
depression and digestion
while stimulating the
abdominal organs.

Pigeon Pose (Kapotasana):
This backbend pose is a bit more advanced than the others; it stretches the hips in both directions and strengthens the back. While not everyone's favourite pose, it does release tension and stress while improving hip flexibility and posture.

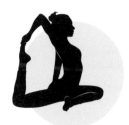

Exercise Tip

To get in touch with our sacral chakra, we need to embrace our inner child. When next exercising, consider activities such as dancing, running, playing with a hula-hoop or skipping rope. Make sure that you're having fun while you're doing it!

MEDITATION AND AFFIRMATIONS

When it comes to meditating for your sacral chakra, it's important to bring creativity into the mix, as this chakra values self-expression above all. Finding your own unique flair may help these meditations really take effect, so while this meditation will help you rebalance and open your sacral chakra, feel free to put your own spin on it. This is especially important if you're looking to nurture or give more love.

 Step One: Sit down on the ground with your legs crossed and your eyes closed. Take three slow, deep breaths to centre yourself.

 Step Two: With your eyes still closed, picture in your mind a bright orange light below your navel. Focus on this light as you place the tips of your index fingers together, and the tips of your thumbs together to form a diamond shape. Your other fingers should also be outstretched. This is called the Trimurta Mudra, which nurtures emotional balance while promoting change.

Step Three: After a moment, begin the *vam* mantra chant (pronounced "foam"). Continue this for a few minutes as you focus on that orange light.

 Step Four: With each chant, continue to breathe life into your chakra. In your head, ask your chakra "what do you need?". The answer may come to you as a colour, a feeling, a flash of an image or a word. Don't force an answer, but let it come naturally.

 Step Five: When you are ready, slow your breathing and chanting down and open your eyes. You could try journaling your experience and feelings after meditation and take note of how these change over time.

As with meditation, getting creative with affirmations can make them more effective. However, if you're experiencing writer's block, here are some suggestions:

- "I embrace all the pleasure life has to offer me."
- "Creativity flows through me."
- "I attract people who respect me."
- "I embrace my sexuality."
- "I choose joy."
- "I honour myself and I respect myself."

SOLAR PLEXUS CHAKRA

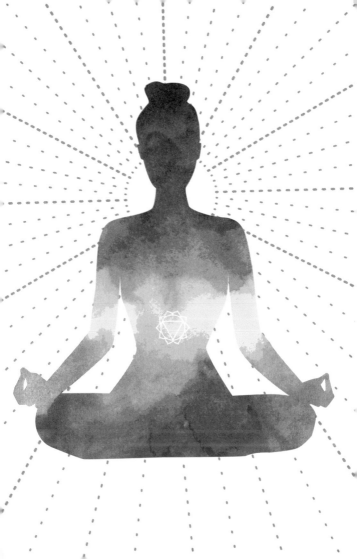

OVERVIEW

As we move from the second chakra to the third, we shift our focus from pleasure to power; the inner child at play becomes a warrior. Located at the base of the ribcage, the solar plexus, or manipura, is focused on our inner power. This chakra rules over our self-confidence, autonomy, willpower and our ability to take action. When balanced, we are ambitious, confident, courageous and independent. We become go-getters with a sense of purpose that makes us want to change the world. When unbalanced, we become deeply insecure and riddled with doubt. We cannot make decisions for ourselves and we passively let others make choices for us.

KEY FACTS

Sanskrit: Manipura – "city of jewels"
Colour: Yellow
Element: Fire
Planet: Mars
Zodiac sign: Aries & Scorpio
Motto: "I can"

MENTAL AND PHYSICAL ASPECTS

"Going with your gut" should be the motto for the solar plexus because it rules over the digestive system, including the stomach; when this chakra is balanced, we trust our decisions and intuition.

Along with our gut, the manipura rules over our intestines, pancreas, upper abdomen, liver, gallbladder, adrenal glands and immune system. It is associated with our digestion and metabolism, so if you start having tummy troubles, a blocked solar plexus may be to blame.

When our solar plexus becomes unbalanced or blocked, it may manifest itself as ulcers or diabetes, or cause issues with the colon, stomach and digestive system. When our chakra is balanced, we feel physically strong, and our stomach and overall health feels good.

For the solar plexus chakra to be aligned, we need to feel we have control over our destiny. The word "power" comes up a lot when discussing the third chakra: not over others, but over ourselves.

Our ambition and drive is vital when considering the third chakra. When balanced, we feel confident about our abilities and our place in the world. We are motivated and have the courage to do what scares us, knowing that it will be worth it in the end. We trust our gut.

Unbalanced, we feel worthless, unable to take control of our lives or to stop ourselves from taking on too many responsibilities. When this chakra is inactive, we can develop an inferiority complex. If overactive, we can become aggressive, controlling and overconfident. To balance this chakra, try to do one thing that scares you each day, even if it's small. By taking risks, we learn to overcome fears and unleash our inner warrior.

IF YOU DOUBT
YOURSELF,
THEN INDEED
YOU STAND ON
SHAKY GROUND.

HENRIK IBSEN

FOOD AND DIET

Our inner warrior needs a healthy diet to achieve our goals and win victories. So how do we feed our third chakra? Let's start off with yellow foods; not only is it the colour of this chakra but it serves as a natural mood enhancer. Foods like corn, pineapple, squash, yellow peppers, lemons, sunflower seeds, camomile tea and yellow curry are excellent choices to refuel with.

Since the solar plexus is ruled by the digestive system, it's important to have complex carbohydrates in your diet as they are a terrific source of fibre and energy. Foods like oats, beans, brown rice, rye bread, spelt and sprouted grains are ideal if you have a blocked solar plexus. This chakra is ruled by the element of fire, so feel free to add some spices like ginger and turmeric for an added kick.

CRYSTALS

Crystals that are associated with the solar plexus chakra, and help heal, clean and stimulate it, include:

Agate: stability, protection and emotional connection.
Bloodstone: creativity, grounding and protection.
Citrine: joy, creativity and abundance.
Golden Healer Lemurian: wisdom, natural gifts and grace.
Honey Calcite: motivation, support and personal power.
Pyrite: personal growth, confidence and passion.
Rutilated Quartz: clarity, energy and awareness.
Yellow Fluorite: unity, intellect and intelligence.
Yellow Jasper: happiness, clarity and self-confidence.

Use these crystals during meditation, when you are feeling self-doubt or are low on confidence. Keep the energy with you throughout the day by attaching one to a keychain, or by placing them by your bedside at night.

ESSENTIAL OILS

Here are a few essential oils that help open the solar plexus chakra and promote feelings of confidence:

Camomile: calmness, inner peace, spiritual awareness, sleep, love and comfort.

Cinnamon: protection, prosperity, happiness, assurance and self-love.

Eucalyptus: balance, concentration, healing, visions and stimulation.

Frankincense: enlightenment, inspiration, luck, protection and introspection.

Juniper Berry: organization, clear thinking, energy, renewal and action.

Lemon: willpower, energy, focus, encouragement and rejuvenation.

Lemongrass: balance, calm, uplifting energy, love and psychic intuition.

Tip: Add a few drops of distilled essential oil to massage lotion and gently rub it into your stomach after a hard day (camomile, eucalyptus or lemongrass work well). If you need some extra courage, apply a few drops of frankincense or lemon oil to your wrists and throat.

I AM NOT AFRAID
OF STORMS, FOR
I'M LEARNING
HOW TO SAIL
MY SHIP.

LOUISA MAY ALCOTT

YOGA POSES

For the solar plexus, it's beneficial to practise yoga poses that build strength and help you burn energy. The solar plexus is our "inner warrior", so we've recommended poses to keep your body feeling fit and healthy. Any pose that helps build confidence during yoga is good (especially for beginners), but here are some to try out:

Cat Pose (Marjaryasana): This backbend pose is ideal for beginners due to its simplicity. This pose helps stretch the upper back and calms the mind, plus it's a very soothing way to start your yoga routine.

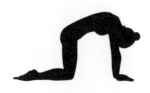

Cobra Pose (Bhujangasana): The name of this pose might have you thinking you need to coil your entire body, but this backbend is much simpler than many other poses. Cobra offers a serious stretch down the front of your body, as well as strengthening your arms. While you may not be exerting much energy, your solar plexus will be gaining a lot of positive energy from this pose.

Boat Pose (Navasana): Boat pose is incredibly effective at strengthening abdominal muscles, but you may struggle to keep from tipping over. However, the rewards are significant as navasana brings power to the solar plexus and puts a fire in your belly. It also stimulates the kidneys and intestines, while improving digestion.

Plank Pose (Kumbhakasana): This pose is common in most workouts as it keeps the energy flowing throughout the body. However, it can become quite intense if you do it for an extended period of time. Plank pose builds strength, is energizing, improves posture and digestion, and strengthens your willpower. If you can be in plank pose for a solid minute, you can do anything!

Exercise Tip

Taking a martial arts class can help unleash your inner warrior as well as build strength, balance and confidence. It may help you take a step out of your comfort zone, which is also great for building up your solar plexus.

MEDITATION AND AFFIRMATIONS

If you've found that your solar plexus has become blocked or overstimulated, here is an easy meditation to do to get it back to a balanced state.

 Step One: Sit down with your legs crossed on the floor.

 Step Two: Close your eyes and take slow, deep breaths until you become fully relaxed.

 Step Three: Place your hands between your heart and your stomach with the palms touching and the thumbs crossed over one another. Cross over all other fingers besides the index fingers, which should be pointing downwards. This is called the Ksepana Mudra and it is meant to relieve tension and improve clarity.

 Step Four: In a low, soft voice, start chanting the *ram* mantra (pronounced "rama"). While doing this, use your mind's eye to visualize yourself achieving your goals. Maybe you see yourself as the CEO of a company, or winning a competition. Whatever it is, visualize how good it would feel to achieve that goal.

 Step Five: When you feel ready, slow your chanting and open your eyes. Take a moment to ground yourself before getting up.

For an added boost, meditate with one of the crystals mentioned on page 51, or set up an oil diffuser containing one of the essential oils listed in the section on page 52.

While you're doing your meditation, or if you just need a little pick me up, here are some affirmations you can repeat to yourself for a boost of confidence:

- "I feel my power."
- "I have everything I need to succeed."
- "I am motivated to pursue my true purpose."
- "I am the captain of my destiny."
- "My desires are within my grasp."
- "I find satisfaction in the life I live."
- "I know my worth."

HEART
CHAKRA

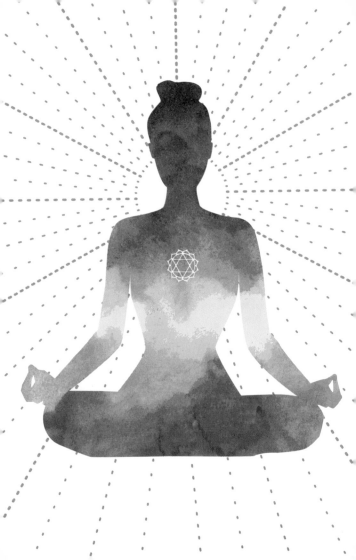

OVERVIEW

As you may have guessed by the name, the heart chakra, or anahata, is all about love and everything that comes along with it: compassion, empathy, kindness, respect, understanding and forgiveness. It's about the connections we have with others, but also with ourselves. The heart chakra reminds us that no one person is an island; we need each other to survive and it's those bonds that give us life. When this chakra is balanced, we are joyful and able to accept love from others and ourselves. When out of balance, we become jealous, bitter and emotionally wounded. However, we are able to move past old wounds through forgiveness, gratitude and love.

KEY FACTS

Sanskrit: Anahata – "unhurt"

Colour: Green

Element: Air

Planet: Venus

Zodiac sign: Taurus & Libra

Motto: "I love"

MENTAL AND PHYSICAL ASPECTS

Located in the centre of the chest, anahata deals with all matters of the heart. Along with ruling the heart, this chakra influences the lungs, thymus gland, oesophagus, circulatory system, arms and hands.

When anahata gets out of balance, some people see it manifest physically through chest pains, poor blood pressure, bronchitis, asthma, pneumonia or a weakened immune system. It's important to take care of your heart health early in life to keep your chakra clear and aligned with the rest of the body.

To really balance your heart chakra you must be kind to your body and take good care of it. Feeding it, nurturing it and making sure it gets enough sleep are great steps, but you must also ensure you're checking in with your mental well-being. You can't take care of anyone else if you're not taking care of yourself.

The heart chakra rules over love in all forms: romantic, familial, platonic and, most importantly, self-love. All relationships can teach us how to give and receive love, but if you don't have a strong connection to yourself, it becomes challenging to maintain strong connections with other people.

When the heart chakra is balanced, we feel loving towards ourselves and others. We are empathic and treat people with kindness, care and respect. We become warm and compassionate, always willing to lend a hand.

When the heart chakra is unbalanced, we feel unloved and unlovable. If blocked, it can manifest into self-pity and depression, making us become needy, clingy and hypercritical. Moreover, an overactive anahata can lead to feelings of entitlement, jealousy, and bitterness. Remember to take care of yourself and ask others for help when needed.

THE HIGHEST
FORMS OF
UNDERSTANDING
WE CAN ACHIEVE
ARE LAUGHTER
AND HUMAN
COMPASSION.

RICHARD FEYNMAN

FOOD AND DIET

As the old saying goes "the best way to a person's heart is through their stomach", so feeding our heart chakra is a good way to open and heal it. Give your heart chakra leafy vegetables like spinach, kale, dandelion greens and cabbage. Other green foods also associated with this chakra are broccoli, cauliflower, celery, basil, thyme, coriander, parsley, cucumber, courgette, avocado, lime, mint, peas, kiwi, green apples and guava. Superfoods like barley, spirulina and chlorella are also good options when feeding your chakra, and green and matcha tea is soothing. If in doubt, a good soup can bring a great deal of comfort, for both you and someone you love.

CRYSTALS

Crystals that are associated with the heart chakra, and help heal, clean and stimulate it include:

Amazonite: soothing energies, balance and trust.
Aventurine: good fortune, opportunity and confidence.
Emerald: success, love and hope.
Garnet: energy, health and romance.
Jade: wisdom, success and abundance.
Malachite: protection, balance and transformation.
Moss Agate: nature, new beginnings and forgiveness.
Peridot: happiness, protection and abundance.
Rose Quartz: healing of any relationship, self-love and emotional balance.

Wear any of these crystals as a pendant around your neck. Having them touch your heart will power anahata. It's also a good idea to meditate with your crystals in the morning to start your day off right.

ESSENTIAL OILS

Here are a few essential oils that help open the heart chakra and promote feelings of self-love and inner peace:

Cypress: harmony, inner peace, wisdom, comfort and trust.

Jasmine: dream, spirits, compassion, money and purpose.

Lavender: restoration, happiness, love, peace and healing.

Lemon Balm: relaxing energies, forgiveness, love and clarity.

Palmarosa: enthusiasm, loyalty, love, healing and gentleness.

Rose: happiness, love, contentment, patience and comfort.

Yarrow: harmony, intuition, love, courage and friendships.

Tip: Place the distilled oil on your breast bone when you want to get to the heart of specific issues. Or, if you want to get sensual with your lover, ask them to rub some massage lotion mixed with a few drops of oil onto your back and see how things progress.

IS THERE ONE WORD WHICH MAY SERVE AS A RULE OF PRACTICE FOR ALL ONE'S LIFE? IS NOT RECIPROCITY SUCH A WORD?

CONFUCIUS

YOGA POSES

For the heart chakra, it's very important to open the chest and breathe deeply to stimulate the lungs. In fact, it's good to take slow, deep breaths before doing any exercise, the added benefit being that it builds upper body strength.

Mountain Pose (Tadasana): While this looks like a simple standing pose, don't be fooled; a lot of energy and focus is required to pull this one off. If done correctly, mountain pose will open up your chest and unblock your heart chakra. It also increases flexibility in the back and stimulates energy through the rest of your routine.

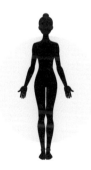

Upward-Facing Dog (Urdhva Mukha Svanasana): Upward-facing dog is a backbend pose similar to cobra, but is more energizing as it opens your chest and strengthens your back and arms for better posture. It also stimulates your abdominal organs and is good for people with asthma.

Camel Pose (Ustrasana): A deep backbend that opens the chest and shoulders to relieve tension in the spine and promote flexibility. It also increases energy flow and improves circulation in the lungs while lowering blood pressure. Make sure you remember to breathe and take your time with this pose.

Wild Thing (Camatkarasana): One translation of camatkarasana means "the ecstatic unfolding of the enraptured heart". This *very* wild pose opens the chest as you bend over backwards to reach for the sky. Not only does this open your heart chakra, it strengthens your arms and legs while increasing back flexibility.

Exercise Tip

Activities such as push-ups and swimming are also great for your heart chakra as they exercise your chest muscles. Don't forget to take a moment to relax and take care of yourself after an intense workout – it's an act of self-love.

MEDITATION AND AFFIRMATIONS

If you feel your anahata is blocked, overactive or not aligned with the rest of your chakras, here's a simple meditation to try:

 Step One: Find a comfortable and quiet place; you can either sit with your legs crossed or lie on your back for this meditation. Close your eyes and focus on your breathing. Listen to your heartbeat.

 Step Two: Place your hands in front of your heart with both of your little fingers and thumbs touching, and the heel of your palms pressed together. Your other fingers should be stretched upward to form a lotus shape. This is called the Padma Mudra.

 Step Three: Visualize a small green light above your heart. Think about all the times you've given and received love in your life, or the type of love you want to bring into your life. As you recall these moments and allow yourself to immerse in them, imagine the light getting bigger and brighter until it fills up the whole space in your mind.

Step Four: Chant the *yam* mantra (pronounced "yum") in one long low voice, coming deep from your lungs.

Step Five: When you're ready, take a few deep breaths before opening your eyes again.

Remember, meditation is a type of self-care, so take as long as you need with your practice.

The best thing you can do to help open, balance or heal your heart chakra is to speak kind words to yourself. Anahata is nourished on words of affirmation, more than any other chakra. Here are a few phrases to say to be a little kinder to yourself:

- "I love who I am and I love who I am becoming."

- "I welcome love into my life."

- "I forgive others; I forgive myself."

- "Love is attracted to me."

- "I create supportive, loving relationships in my life."

- "I am healing every day."

- "I am open to kindness."

THROAT
CHAKRA

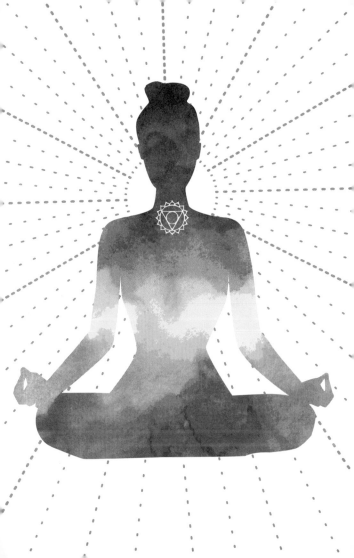

OVERVIEW

The throat chakra, or vishuddha, speaks for us and everything we believe in. It is responsible for determining how we express ourselves and our personal truths. Located at the centre of the neck, the throat chakra focuses our ability to communicate clearly, vocalize our needs and share our innermost selves with the world. When balanced, we can articulate our thoughts, feelings and ideas with honesty and assertiveness. If the throat chakra is unbalanced, it becomes difficult to know when and how to verbalize our opinions, resulting in miscommunication.

KEY FACTS

Sanskrit: Vishuddha – "especially pure"
Colour: Blue
Element: Sound
Planet: Mercury
Zodiac sign: Gemini & Virgo
Motto: "I speak"

MENTAL AND PHYSICAL ASPECTS

It's not difficult to guess what parts of the body vishuddha rules over. However, besides the throat and neck, this chakra is responsible for the vocal cords, mouth, tongue, teeth, shoulders, lips, ears and lymphatic system. If it helps you talk or listen, it's probably run by the throat chakra.

When out of alignment, we tend to suffer from sore throats and lingering coughs that won't go away. It can also result in gum and teeth issues, hearing loss, voice problems and a stiff neck. Grinding your teeth, biting your lip until it bleeds, or having a constant sore throat, are all ways this chakra responds to stress.

One way to heal vishuddha is to sing, even if you're bad at it. Let go of self-judgement and put on a solo concert for an audience of one – you'll find it very enjoyable and your throat chakra will benefit from it.

The throat chakra rules over the expression of our desires, needs, beliefs and creativity as well as dealing with issues of self-worth and responsibility. The truth is vital to vishuddha. When we are not speaking our truth, we are not living our most authentic life. However, balance is key. While it's important to say what we feel, we must take other people's feelings into account. Listening to others helps build connections to the people around us and increases our knowledge and understanding.

The throat chakra becomes blocked when we cannot express ourselves through regular means of communication, such as speaking or writing. We are timid, dependent on others, and fearful of public speaking. When we live a lie, hide the truth, or stay silent on important issues, our chakra becomes unbalanced. When overactive, we talk too much and interrupt others. We gossip, lie and are unable to keep important secrets. To balance this chakra, we must find our voice.

I FOUND I COULD
SAY THINGS WITH
COLOUR AND
SHAPES THAT I
COULDN'T SAY
ANY OTHER WAY
- THINGS I HAD
NO WORDS FOR.

GEORGIA O'KEEFFE

FOOD AND DIET

It's important to feed your chakra the right foods, but in this case, liquids play a more important role as they're easier on the throat. If you need to nurture your chakra, reach for things like herbal teas with honey, coconut water, bone broth, lemon water and syrup.

If it's food that you're craving, blue foods such as blueberries and blackberries are great options. However, as there aren't many blue foods in nature, fruits from the tree, like apples, pears, oranges, peaches, apricots and plums, are often used to feed this chakra. Why tree fruits? Fruits only fall from the tree when they are ripe and ready, making them an entirely authentic source of nourishment.

Lastly, stay away from dairy when trying to balance this chakra, because it can congest your throat and sinuses if you have too much.

CRYSTALS

Crystals that are associated with the throat chakra, and help heal, clean and stimulate it include:

Angelite: creativity, guidance and faith.
Aquamarine: stress relief, meditation and good fortune.
Blue Lace Agate: inner stability, steadiness and maturity.
Blue Topaz: strength, communication and intelligence.
Celestite: sharp mental ability, psychic ability and calmness.
Lapis Lazuli: truth, wisdom and learning.
Sapphire: wisdom, prophecy and royalty.
Sodalite: self-expression, truth and intuition.
Turquoise: health, protection and wisdom.

Wear a choker necklace with one of these crystals to have it close to your throat chakra, or meditate with it before a big confrontation where you'll need to speak your truth. Keep a crystal at your desk at work (especially by your phone or laptop) for clear communication and positive interactions with others.

ESSENTIAL OILS

Here are a few essential oils that help open the throat chakra as well as promoting self-expression and improving communication:

Basil: cheerfulness, integrity, trust, wealth and awareness of reality.

Coriander: creativity, enthusiasm, imagination, optimism and compassion.

Fennel: clarity, perseverance, protection, healing and grounding.

Myrrh: acceptance, forgiveness, peace and uplifting energies.

Peppermint: concentration, regeneration, vibrancy and calmness.

Spruce: self-expression, communication, creativity, focus and cleansing energies.

Vanilla: relaxation, happiness, mental strength, empowerment and good luck.

Tip: Dab perfume or body spray containing these essential oils on the pulse points of your neck to influence your throat chakra. This will make it easier to express yourself effectively.

THY VOICE IS A CELESTIAL MELODY.

HENRY WADSWORTH LONGFELLOW

YOGA POSES

Neck flexibility is a must for any healthy throat chakra. A strong, healthy neck is good for our vocal cords and our ability to speak the truth on important subjects. Here are some poses for you to try:

Warrior II (Virabhadrasana II): The sequel to Warrior I on page 24, this standing pose is probably one of the most recognizable, and it's easy to learn. Make sure your neck is as straight as possible; this improves circulation and respiration while opening your lungs. It also helps balance your body while empowering your mind.

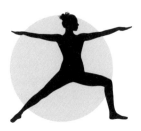

Fish Pose (Matsyasana): This is a great position for those needing to channel a more relaxing energy. This restorative backbend opens the throat chakra by stretching the neck, while encouraging flexibility in the upper spine and shoulders.

Plough Pose (Halasana): An inversion pose, plough encourages a straight neck as the rest of the body bends in the other direction. Despite how uncomfortable it may appear, plough pose calms the mind and reduces stress while stretching out the back and shoulders. It also stimulates the abdominal organs and thyroid gland.

Supported Shoulder Stand (Salamba Sarvangasana): Typically done after plough pose, this is another calming inversion pose that feels better than it looks. It loosens up the neck and shoulders while boosting blood flow in the upper body. It also stimulates the thyroid while calming the mind.

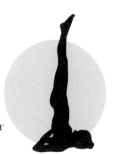

Exercise Tip

While many people don't think singing counts as exercise, it's a great way to improve lung health, strengthen your vocal cords, and get the air moving throughout your body. When you need to give your throat chakra a boost, start chanting during meditation, or sing your favourite song. Don't worry about whether you're a good singer or not – just let it out!

MEDITATION AND AFFIRMATIONS

If you feel your throat chakra needs realigning, here is a simple way to find your voice again through meditation.

 Step One: Go into a room and either sit or stand with your back completely straight.

 Step Two: When you are ready, close your eyes and begin focusing on your breathing. Inhale deeply at whatever pace you feel comfortable with.

 Step Three: Place your hands in front of you with the palms facing up. Lay one hand on top of the other with the tips of your fingers pointing in opposite directions. Touch the tip of your thumbs to make a circle. This is called the Dhyana Mudra, used for reflection and calming energy. Take a large breath in and out of the body and clear your throat.

 Step Four: When you're ready, start humming; this is known as the *ham* mantra. While humming, visualize a blue light appearing around the centre of your neck. Watch it get brighter the more you hum.

 Step Five: Slow down your humming until your voice trails off naturally. Take a moment to steady yourself before opening your eyes again.

Tip: To bring more sound to your meditation, try using a singing bowl. The vibrations of the deep tones promote relaxation and harmonize with your body.

Words are important, especially for your throat chakra. Here are some affirmations to repeat while meditating to help balance the chakra:

- "I speak my truth with power."
- "My voice gets stronger every day."
- "I communicate clearly and honestly."
- "I am open to new opinions."
- "I live authentically."
- "I have integrity."
- "I know when to listen and when to speak."

THIRD EYE CHAKRA

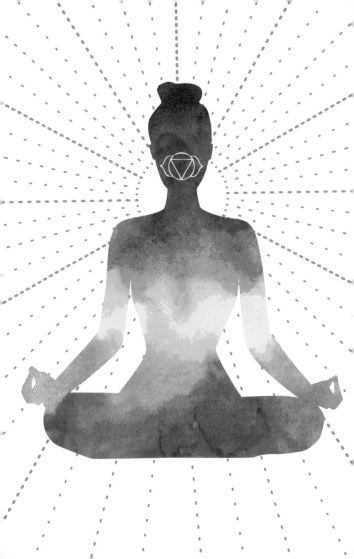

OVERVIEW

This chakra is known by many names – the sixth sense, primal instinct, clairvoyance – but we'll stick to its commonly recognized name: the third eye, or ajna. Located on the brow between your two physical eyes, the third eye allows you to see what is hidden from physical perception. It deals with our insight, intuition and wisdom. If you've ever had a hunch, like getting goosebumps before receiving bad news or "guessing" the correct answer, then you've already experienced your third eye at work. When it's balanced, we trust our intuition and are open to changes. When unbalanced, we feel uncertain, blinded by the opinions of others.

KEY FACTS

Sanskrit: Ajna – "command"
Colour: Indigo
Element: Light
Planet: Sun & moon
Zodiac sign: Leo & Cancer
Motto: "I see"

MENTAL AND PHYSICAL ASPECTS

The third eye chakra not only deals with our hidden eye, but our two physical eyes as well. It rules over our nose, sinuses, brain, nervous system and the pituitary gland. When this chakra is in balance, we sleep well, our vision and sense of smell are strong and our memory is sharp.

However, when ajna is unbalanced, it can manifest into eye pain, dry eyes, headaches and migraines, high blood pressure, and problems with vision, the sinuses and the spine. We are unable to sleep properly and can experience issues with brain fog and lapses in memory.

Peaceful activities like yoga, qigong or swimming are great at unblocking the third eye chakra. It's also good to wear blue-light-blocking glasses when working on your computer or tablet for long periods of time to prevent eye strain.

Ajna rules over our imagination, memory, clairvoyance and psychic wisdom. It is how we perceive the spiritual world. The third eye chakra plays an important role in how we view ourselves, our visions for the future, and the truth.

When the third eye is open, we are intuitive, charismatic, meditative, wise and decisive, and we know our value and purpose in life. We tend to make the right decisions without thinking about it because we are guided by our instincts, which can see what we physically can't.

When this chakra is blocked, we are afraid of the future and feel as though life is meaningless. We become lost, depressed, spaced out and unsure of who we truly are. When this chakra is overactive, we're easily influenced by delusions and fantasy – we become paranoid, doubtful, and unaware of what's going on around us.

Using tarot cards, or other forms of divination, is a great way to open your third eye, because it strengthens your intuition.

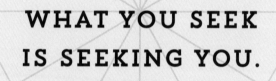

WHAT YOU SEEK
IS SEEKING YOU.

RUMI

FOOD AND DIET

If you want your third eye to have 20/20 vision, you will need to feed it the right foods. Start by eating foods with blue to purple hues like blueberries, blackberries, purple grapes, aubergine, poppy seeds, purple kale and purple sweet potatoes.

While not purple, cocoa is great to have in your diet because it contains antioxidants that cause a release of serotonin in the brain, making you feel happy.

It's also important to add foods rich in omega-3 to your diet, including salmon, walnut, chia seeds and avocado, for boosting brainpower.

CRYSTALS

Crystals that are associated with the third eye chakra, and help heal, clean and stimulate it include:

Charoite: connection, insight and generosity.
Fluorite: peace, clarity and serenity.
Iolite: vision, confidence and creativity.
Labradorite: curiosity, magic and spiritual guidance.
Lapis Lazuli: truth, wisdom and learning.
Star Sapphire: wisdom, success and analytical ability.
Sugilite: psychic protection, stability and mental growth.
Tanzanite: truth, compassion and harmony.
Unakite: positivity, stress relief and kindness.

Sleep with any of these crystals under your pillow to awaken your psychic intuition through dreams. If meditating lying down, place the crystal on your forehead, right between your eyebrows, to help open the chakra.

ESSENTIAL OILS

Here are a few essential oils that help open the third eye chakra and encourage intuition, decision-making and the skill to see things hidden from the naked eye:

Almond: wisdom, prosperity, magic, spirituality and luck.

Bay Laurel: confidence, creativity, direction and inspiration.

Carrot Seed: grounding energy, fertility, improved vision, harmony and spiritual insight.

Clary Sage: balance, calm, tranquility, wisdom and restoration.

Helichrysum: imagination, guidance, spirituality, compassion and understanding.

Marjoram: calm, perseverance, happiness, health and protection.

Mugwort: relaxation, tranquility, protection, magic and vivid dreams.

Tip: Place a drop of essential oil or anointing oil between the eyebrows to open or unblock the third eye. You can also place essential oils in a diffuser and breathe in the good vibes.

TRUST THE
DREAMS, FOR IN
THEM IS HIDDEN
THE GATE TO
ETERNITY.

KAHLIL GIBRAN

YOGA POSES

You may be wondering, "How do I work out my third eye? I can't even see it!" Well, it's all about perspective and looking at things from all angles, even the things that are hidden from the naked eye. Trying lots of different poses that aren't too complicated will allow you to think; doing them with your eyes closed or blindfolded will really make use of ajna. Here are some suggestions for you to try:

Child's Pose (Balasana): This is a very basic pose that usually comes at the beginning of yoga routines. It stimulates the third eye because the forehead is physically touching the ground. It allows a moment of mental concentration before getting started, and is very relaxing.

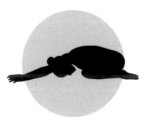

Legs Up the Wall Pose (Viparita Karani): This relaxing and restorative pose doesn't require a lot of twists and turns – all you need is a wall. This pose relaxes the body and opens the third eye chakra while allowing you to see things from a different point of view.

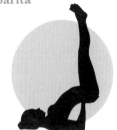

Standing Forward Bend (Uttanasana): This simple pose offers a host of benefits. It releases tension in the body while stretching the lower back, hamstrings, glutes and hips while also stimulating blood flow towards the third eye.

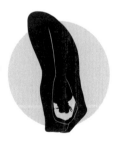

Downward-Facing Dog (Adho Mukha Svanasana): One of the most famous yoga poses, downward-facing dog is one of the first positions you learn when starting yoga. This forward bend strengthens the legs, wrists and hips, as well as increasing circulation to your third eye. It also helps relieve headaches while making you more alert and focused.

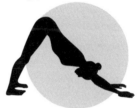

Exercise Tip

Mental exercises – such as puzzles, journaling, shuffling tarot cards, or playing guessing games – test and strengthen your third eye. You don't need to work your whole body in order to work your chakra.

MEDITATION AND AFFIRMATIONS

Meditation is key for opening and strengthening your third eye chakra. It will help you gain insight into other realms and may provide visions of the future. Here is a simple way to get that eye open. Preferably, do this one before bed.

 Step One: Perform your nightly routine, but place a pen and a pad of paper by your bedside before getting into bed and turning the lights off.

 Step Two: Close your eyes and start taking deep breaths; in through your nose and out through your mouth. As you're doing this, visualize an indigo light that gets bigger each time you exhale.

 Step Three: Place your hands together on the lower part of your chest and let the tips of your middle fingers meet. Curl your other fingers, tucking them into your palms so the backs of the fingers touch. Press the tips of your thumbs together, forming a kind of heart shape. This is called the Kalesvara Mudra and is used to promote optimism.

Step Four: In a low, quiet voice, chant the *sham* mantra (pronounced "shum"). If you are unable to speak out loud, chant it in your head. Continue to chant until you feel sleepy, then allow yourself to drift off.

 Step Five: When you wake up the next morning, record any dreams and try to decode their meaning.

Here are some affirmations to repeat to yourself to help open your third eye chakra:

- "I trust my intuition."

- "I am guided by my higher consciousness."

- "I nurture my spirit."

- "I forgive the past, I learn from the past."

- "I trust that I'm being guided down the right path for me."

- "I am open to inspiration and bliss."

- "Everything that is happening to me is for my highest good."

CROWN
CHAKRA

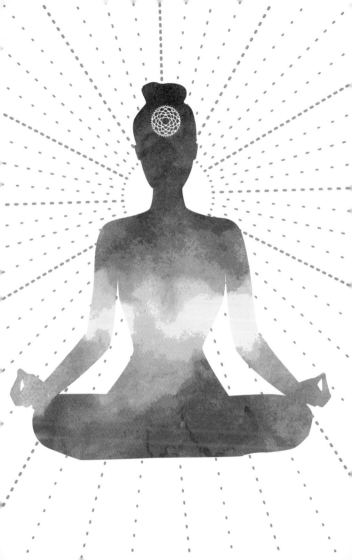

OVERVIEW

We've reached the final chakra: the crown, or sahasrara. Our journey to enlightenment is nearly complete. Located on the very top of the head, the crown chakra connects us to the Divine. The root chakra brought us closer to the earth, but the crown chakra sets free the limitless possibilities that the world has to offer. When it's balanced, our minds are open and we are guided by a force greater than ourselves. We see past self-limiting beliefs and material desires. Out of balance, we feel lost and without a sense of purpose. It may take a person many years to open the crown chakra, but it is worth the journey.

KEY FACTS

Sanskrit: Sahasrara – "lotus of a thousand petals"
Colour: Violet/white
Element: Thought
Planet: Transcendence
Zodiac sign: Transcendence
Motto: "I know"

MENTAL AND PHYSICAL ASPECTS

Sahasrara rules over the upper part of our brain, the pineal gland, the cerebral cortex, the central nervous system and the skin. These parts of the body do an essential job to keep us alive; we could not live without them, yet we hardly ever consider them. They are automatic, keeping our bodies moving without our command, just like the universe guiding us through life without us having to think about it.

When this chakra is out of alignment, it can manifest physically in headaches, chronic fatigue, weakening of the muscular system, memory problems, neurological disorders, nerve pain, mental fog, skin rashes, insomnia and depression.

To realign the crown chakra, try developing a meditation routine, setting intentions, or going for silent walks by yourself to clear your head and get in touch with nature. Volunteer work also does the body and the chakra good.

The crown chakra deals with our beliefs about the world we live in and the systems around us. Our pre-existing beliefs about belonging in our society can limit our ability to grow, whereas the crown chakra wants us to develop spiritually, mentally and emotionally. There is more to the universe than our little world. Only when we let go of expectations can we truly gain enlightenment.

When the crown chakra is balanced, we are connected to our higher self, or inner sage, and are receptive to the inner and outer beauty of the world. We are wise, compassionate and spiritually connected. We are content.

When sahasrara is overactive, we think that we *are* Divine, acting as prophets or obsessed with religion and spirituality. We become desperate for attention. When the crown chakra is blocked or inactive, we are misunderstood, joyless and depressed. To help balance this chakra, practise daily gratitude.

PATIENCE IS THE COMPANION OF WISDOM.

SAINT AUGUSTINE

FOOD AND DIET

Feeding the crown chakra is tricky, mainly as it doesn't require any food. Sahasrara is focused on our enlightenment, so we need to nourish our spirit rather than our physical body, which means fasting. Many religions and spiritual practices encourage fasting to gain spiritual awareness and become closer to the divine. If you do intend on fasting, it's important to stay hydrated, so drink plenty of water or herbal teas, like peppermint or ginger.

However, if you cannot fast for whatever reason, try to keep your diet as clean as possible, meaning no processed foods of any kind. You can also eat foods that are clear, white or translucent, like coconuts, mushrooms, garlic and potatoes.

CRYSTALS

Crystals that are associated with the crown chakra, and help heal, clean and stimulate it include:

Amethyst: trust, intuition and spirituality.
Beryl: protection, relief and spiritual healing.
Clear Quartz: clarity, focus and visualization.
Diamond: strength, positivity and fortitude.
Howlite: emotional expression, higher consciousness and open-mindedness.
Milky Quartz: healing, confidence and relaxation.
Moonstone: stability, spirituality and sensuality.
Opal: optimism, good luck and reflection.
Selenite: clarity, purifying and recharging.

These crystals are great for meditating, especially when your energy is low or you are in need of spiritual guidance. They help shift your energy from negative to positive, so keep them close if you're having a particularly stressful day. Or, if you want to go the extra mile, wear a crown of these crystals.

ESSENTIAL OILS

Here are a few essential oils that help to open the crown chakra and to promote feelings of spirituality and encourage a connection to your higher consciousness:

Camphor: inner healing, freedom, uplifting energies, divinity and rebirth.

Gotu Kola: intelligence, clarity, joy, longevity and connection.

Lime: creativity, alertness, spiritual strength, protection and zest for life.

Lotus: regeneration, faith, freedom, growth and karma.

Palo Santo: cleansing energy, tranquility, spirituality, balance and communication with other worlds.

Pine: spiritual direction, mindfulness, simplicity, protection and healing.

Spikenard: emotional balance, rest, courage, forgiveness and luck.

Tip: The best way to benefit from these essential oils is to use them in a diffuser. The scent and energy will surround you, allowing you to breathe in their powers. It's especially useful when meditating.

BEFORE ENLIGHTENMENT: CHOP WOOD, CARRY WATER. AFTER ENLIGHTENMENT: CHOP WOOD, CARRY WATER.

ZEN BUDDHIST PROVERB

YOGA POSES

Sahasrara is the highest of the chakras, located just above our head, so many of the yoga poses we do should be concentrated on that area. The yoga poses you choose for the crown chakra should also focus on calming your body, stimulating your mind and keeping your energy balanced overall. Here are a few suggestions to get started:

Lotus Pose (Padmasana): This seated yoga pose is meant to help centre your mind, taking you to your higher self. Lotus pose stabilizes your core and stimulates the spine as you take in deep breaths, which can calm your body.

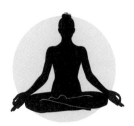

Half-Moon Pose (Ardha Chandrasana): This pose is particularly challenging as you must use all of your muscles and limbs to stay balanced, requiring a lot of concentration and focus. Half-moon pose strengthens your legs while giving your crown chakra energy.

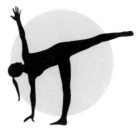

Headstand (Salamba Sirsasana): The grand finale! This inversion pose is only for the most experienced yogis. This position brings the blood flow directly to your crown chakra and really gives it some energy. Large amounts of focus will be needed to keep you in this position, but it will help clear your mind as old thoughts leave your body.

Corpse Pose (Savasana): Don't let the name scare you; this is an easy pose to do at the end of most yoga practices – you are just lying down. But how does lying down benefit your crown chakra? The answer is that it helps you become grounded and centred so you can effectively practise meditation and observe how your yoga session made you feel.

Exercise Tip

Just as it's important to establish a workout routine, it's also important to establish a solid meditative practice during which you set your intentions and clear your mind of all negative thoughts. Only when the body and mind are in balance can we truly be happy and healthy.

MEDITATION AND AFFIRMATIONS

Meditation is crucial to the health and balance of the crown chakra because it's how we connect with our higher self. If you wish to open your crown chakra, try this meditation:

 Step One: Sit down with your legs crossed. Take a few deep breaths in and out to ground yourself.

 Step Two: In your mind's eye, begin to visualize a bright violet light above you. Watch as it gets bigger and smaller again with each breath.

 Step Three: Hold your hands high above your head with the tips of your fingers touching. Stretch your thumbs and little fingers out to the side so that your hands form a triangle shape. This is called the Hakini Mudra.

 Step Four: In your mind, recite everything you're grateful for in that moment. It doesn't have to be anything big; it can be something small like "I saw a beautiful flower on the way to work". You can list as many items as you wish.

Step Five: Give a low *om* mantra. The longer your chant, the closer the violet light comes until it engulfs you. Take a moment to absorb that energy.

 Step Six: After you soak in the energy from the light, take a moment to steady your breath and open your eyes. Stay where you are for a moment before standing up and going about your day.

For some extra help, here are some affirmations to repeat to yourself during the day or during your meditation:

- "Life will bring me many lessons and wonders today."
- "I connect with my higher self."
- "I am aware and centred."
- "I surrender to my spiritual will."
- "I am tuned to the divine energy around me."
- "I am mindful."
- "I release what I do not need."

OTHER CHAKRAS

As mentioned in the first chapter, there are believed to be up to 114 chakras besides the ones mentioned in this book. These chakras live in various places inside or outside the body. While they are not as popular, each serves its own purpose and improves your overall sense of well-being. Here are just a few examples of other chakras in the chakra system.

EARTH STAR CHAKRA

Also known as the super root chakra, the earth star chakra is located roughly 30 cm below our feet, connecting us to the core of the earth. The earth star chakra works best when we are physically connected to the ground, walking barefoot on soft grass, taking a stroll on the beach, or lying down. By connecting with this chakra, we become grounded, with a strong connection to nature. It gives energy to the other chakras, especially the root, given its closeness. The earth star chakra contains the key to our past lives, ancestral origins and our karma.

SOUL STAR CHAKRA

Also referred to as the "seat of the soul", the soul star chakra is located roughly 30 cm above our crown chakra. It connects our very soul to ultimate enlightenment by sending divine light and love into the universe. When the soul star chakra is in balance, we feel a closer connection to our higher self and are content with life. When unbalanced, we may become confused, aloof and spaced out, and suffer from headaches, paranoia, mental fragility and depression. When this chakra is activated, we rise above our ego and are able to experience happiness, spirituality and wellness more fully as we have nothing holding us back.

BINDU CHAKRA

Also referred to as "moon centre", the bindu chakra is located at the back of the head, between the third eye and the crown chakra. Bindu is a Sanskrit word meaning "point" or "drop". The bindu chakra represents the power of physical and mental healing and promotes inner harmony, mental clarity, and balance between the physical and spiritual body. It also controls consciousness. When balanced, this chakra helps with depression, anxiety and feelings of oppression as well as controlling hunger and improving eyesight.

LALANA CHAKRA

Also known as the talu chakra, this chakra is located at the roof of the mouth and is connected to the throat chakra. It is associated with respect, contentment, self-control, pride, affection and honour. When it is in balance, we know when to pick our battles and how to speak to others respectfully. When out of balance, we become dissatisfied and lack self-control, which in turn generates feelings of sorrow, depression and anxiety.

HRIT CHAKRA

Right below the heart chakra, the hrit chakra represents our spiritual heart and what we wish to manifest. This chakra's function is to absorb energy from the sun and give it to the seven main chakras within the body in order to heal or activate them. When balanced, we have the complete freedom to love unconditionally, show kindness to all beings, and be affectionate and compassionate. We have a high sense of self-worth and feel connected to something bigger than ourselves. When this chakra is unbalanced, we are controlled by our ego and lack freedom. We become manipulative and selfish, unable to express love or affection because we are so disconnected from everything. The hrit chakra is also where we store negative feelings and experiences from our past lives, so if this chakra is blocked, it may be because you are dealing with trauma that you need to work through.

ELBOW CHAKRA

The elbow chakra represents our ability to be flexible in mind, body and soul. It rules over our ability to adapt and harmonize to new situations. When it is in balance, we can move forward from grief, we are open-minded and able to accept whatever life throws at us. When unbalanced, we hold onto grudges, unable to let anything go. We become stubborn and set in our ways, possessive and narrow-minded.

KNEE CHAKRA

Located near the knee, this chakra rules over our sense of power; not over others, but over our own actions and thoughts. When balanced, we feel confident, flexible and are able to go with the flow. When out of balance, we are inflexible, scared, and feel overwhelmed and unsure. To balance this chakra, we must "bend the knee" and surrender to our higher power.

CONCLUSION

Hopefully you have enjoyed learning more about the chakras, and have discovered new ways to open, balance and heal them. We may be at the end of this book, but your journey has just begun! The information in these pages is just the starting point on your path to effective chakra healing. Whatever areas you found most interesting in this book, there is still so much more to learn on your quest for enlightenment.

There is no better way to end this book than by adding one more meditation for you to try. This is for activating all your chakras, putting them in perfect balance.

 Step One: In a quiet room, sit on the floor with your legs crossed and your hands resting gently on your knees. Close your eyes and relax.

 Step Two: Start taking deep breaths; inhale through your nose and exhale through your mouth. Do this for several minutes.

 Step Three: Whenever you're ready, imagine a red glow around the base of your spine, representing your root chakra. Continue to picture it as you curl your toes. When it is at its brightest, move onto your sacral chakra and imagine an orange light below your navel. Continue this for the next five chakras.

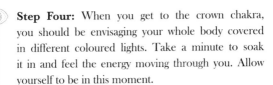

Step Four: When you get to the crown chakra, you should be envisaging your whole body covered in different coloured lights. Take a minute to soak it in and feel the energy moving through you. Allow yourself to be in this moment.

Step Five: When you are ready, slowly open your eyes to the world. Express gratitude to your higher self for allowing this moment.

Be well.

FURTHER READING

Adams, Autumn *The Little Book of Mudra Meditations* (2020, Rockridge Press)

Alcantara, Margarita *Chakra Healing* (2017, Althea)

Carvel, Astrid *The Little Book of Crystals* (2019, Summersdale)

D'Arrigo, Christina *Essential Chakra Yoga* (2020, Rockridge Press)

Dickinson, Ross *The Little Book of World Religions* (2020, Summersdale)

Golding, Sophie *Live Better* (2017, Vie)

Leigh, Amy and Mercree, Chad *A Little Bit of Chakras* (2016, Sterling Ethos)

Mercier, Patricia *The Bible Chakra* (2009, Godsfield Press)

Perrakis, Athena *The Ultimate Guide to Chakras* (2018, Fair Winds)

Saradananda, Swami *Chakra Meditation* (2011, Duncan Baird)

Saradananda, Swami *Mudras for Modern Life* (2015, Watkins Publishing)

Swanberg, Sarah *Aromatherapy for Self-Care* (2020, Rockridge Press)

IMAGE CREDITS

If you're interested in finding out more
about our books, find us on Facebook at
Summersdale Publishers and follow us
on Twitter at **@Summersdale**.

WWW.SUMMERSDALE.COM